PALEO MEAL PREP

Beginners Guide to Meal Prep 4-Weeks of Paleo Diet Recipes (28 Full Days of Paleo Meals)

Olivia Rogers

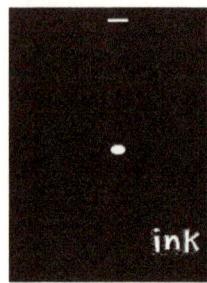

First published in 2019 by Venture Ink Publishing

Copyright © The Menu At Home 2019

All rights reserved.

No part of this book may be reproduced in any form without permission in writing from the author. No part of this publication may be reproduced or transmitted in any form or by any means, mechanic, electronic, photocopying, recording, by any storage or retrieval system, or transmitted by email without the permission in writing from the author and publisher.

Requests to the publisher for permission should be addressed to publishing@ventureink.co

For more information about the contents of this book or questions to the author, please contact Olivia Rogers at olivia@themenuathome.com

Disclaimer

This book provides wellness management information in an informative and educational manner only, with information that is general in nature and that is not specific to you, the reader. The contents of this book are intended to assist you and other readers in your personal wellness efforts. Consult your physician regarding the applicability of any information provided in this book to you.

Nothing in this book should be construed as personal advice or diagnosis, and must not be used in this manner. The information provided about conditions is general in nature. This information does not cover all possible uses, actions, precautions, side-effects, or interactions of medicines, or medical procedures. The information in this book should not be considered as complete and does not cover all diseases, ailments, physical conditions, or their treatment.

You should consult with your physician before beginning any exercise, weight loss, or health care program. This book should not be used in place of a call or visit to a competent health-care professional. You should consult a health care professional before adopting any of the suggestions in this book or before drawing inferences from it.

Any decision regarding treatment and medication for your condition should be made with the advice and consultation of a qualified health care professional. If you have, or suspect you have, a health-care problem, then you should immediately contact a qualified health care professional for treatment.

No Warranties: The author and publisher don't guarantee or warrant the quality, accuracy, completeness, timeliness, appropriateness or suitability of the information in this book, or of any product or services referenced in this book.

The information in this book is provided on an "as is" basis and the author and publisher make no representations or warranties of any kind with respect to this information. This book may contain inaccuracies, typographical errors, or other errors.

Liability Disclaimer: The publisher, author, and other parties involved in the creation, production, provision of information, or delivery of this book specifically disclaim any responsibility, and shall not be held liable for any damages, claims, injuries, losses, liabilities, costs, or obligations including any direct, indirect, special, incidental, or consequences damages (collectively known as "Damages") whatsoever and howsoever caused, arising out of, or in connection with the use or misuse of the site and the information contained within it, whether such Damages arise in contract, tort, negligence, equity, statute law, or by way of other legal theory.

Table of Contents

Disclaimer	3
Who Is This Book For?	7
What Will This Book Teach You?	9
Introduction	11
Getting Started with Meal Prep	13
About the Paleo Diet	17
Week 1	23
Week 2	29
Week 3	37
Week 4	45
Conclusion	51
Final Words	53

Who Is This Book For?

This book is for everyone who wants to follow the Paleo diet but doesn't have the time to cook from scratch.

It's for people who have busy lives and just want a simple and straight forward way to eat healthy and tasty meals.

Eating well isn't easy these days, and if you're dedicated to the Paleo diet, it can be even more complicated.

It means that you can't just grab any food from the fridge or off the shelves at the supermarket, you need to adhere to the guidelines of the diet. And cooking meals that fit these guidelines can take time, particularly if you aren't used to it.

If you're new to the Paleo diet, it might take you time to work out which foods, sauces and recipes suit your new eating plan, and even longer to cook your meals.

But meal prepping can help with that. Doing meal prep will cut down on the amount of time you spend preparing food and cooking meals on a daily basis.

It will mean that, when you get home tired and late, there is a quick and simple meal option in the fridge or freezer waiting for you.

Basically, learning to meal prep will make your life and your meals easier, quicker and healthier.

So you can enjoy an eating plan that suits your health and wellbeing without spending all your free time in the kitchen.

If this sounds good to you, let's get started!

What Will This Book Teach You?

Planning and cooking healthy, delicious meals can be difficult even if you're not on a specific diet. But if you follow the Paleo diet, it can be even more difficult.

This book will help with that. It will teach you how to do meal prep for easy and delicious Paleo meals so you always have a quick and healthy meal waiting in the fridge when you get home.

This will stop you from reaching for an easy option that just doesn't fit with your diet plan.

Doing meal prep may seem as if it would take a lot of time. But in reality, it will save you time on a day to day basis.

It's the perfect option for the days and weeks when you're too busy to think about cooking, but still want to eat foods that are good for you and good for your body.

So whether you have a family, or if you cook for yourself, this book will give you a basic understanding of the Paleo diet.

It will give you 28 days of Paleo recipes along with a detailed description of the prep you need to do for each meal.

Following this meal plan will help you stick to your diet, even on the days when you're tired or busy. And that will help you enjoy all of the health benefits that the Paleo diet has to offer.

So happy prepping and eating!

Introduction

If you have a busy life, don't enjoy cooking after a full day of work, or just want to make it easier to eat according to the Paleo diet, you need to try meal prep.

To put it simply, meal prep is any action you take to prepare your meals ahead of time.

This means you can cook the meals and freeze them or just separate the ingredients for each recipe and store them ready to cook.

That way, when you're ready to eat, you just take the right container out of the fridge or freezer and reheat or cook the prepared ingredients.

Meal prep is particularly good when you're on a particular diet, such as the Paleo diet. Preparing your food ahead of time means you don't have to think about the Paleo rules in the evening when you're tired and just want to eat whatever is easiest.

Doing meal prep means you have the convenience of a TV dinner, but made at home with fresh, unprocessed ingredients. It's the easiest way to make sure that you and your family are eating healthy meals without spending all evening in the kitchen.

There are many different ways to do meal prep depending on how much time you have and how many days you want to prepare for. You can prepare for three days of eating, or go really brave and prepare a week's worth of meals on your prep day.

This book will teach you how to do the latter. It will teach you large recipes that make at least seven meals so you can freeze a couple for later in the week and have some in the fridge ready to reheat immediately. Just make sure you follow the storage guidelines so the meals are still safe to eat after a week.

Meal prepping this way means you basically only have to cook 3 meals a week to have seven days' worth of delicious paleo meals with no trouble or fuss. And that includes breakfasts, lunches and dinners. After your prep day, you won't have to think about any of them.

Getting Started with Meal Prep

Before you actually start prepping your meals, there are a few guidelines you should keep in mind.

These will help make the process smoother and easier, and that will make you more likely to keep doing it!

The most important thing about meal prep is to understand how long you can keep foods in the fridge. This differs depending on the type of food, for example meat doesn't keep very long at all, and whether the food is cooked or not before you store it.

Here are some guidelines for storing food in the fridge:

- If it smells or has something growing on it, ignore all the following advice and throw it out immediately.

- Store everything in airtight containers.

- If stored in an airtight container, cut vegetables will keep between 2 and 4 days depending on the type of vegetable.

- Cooked eggs will last about 7 days in the fridge.

- Make sure you choose vegetables that won't wilt if you're keeping them in the fridge such as potatoes, sweet potatoes, cauliflower and carrots.

- Cooked meat will keep in the fridge for 3-4 days. Any longer than that and you need to freeze it.

- As for uncooked meat, make sure you follow the expiration date on the packet.

- Make sure that when you reheat food, it's steaming all the way through. The food should be above 70 degrees when you're done reheating.

- Never reheat food more than once. Store your meals in separate containers so you can reheat exactly the amount you need.

A Guide to Freezing

The biggest benefit of prepping is that you have quick and easy meals already in the fridge and ready to eat. But this means that you have to eat the meals before they go bad.

There are different guidelines you need to follow for food safety and freshness. These are:

- Most frozen meals can be kept for 3-6 months in the freezer.

- Before freezing, make sure you leave a little room at the top of the container so the food can expand.

- When cooking frozen meals, make sure you heat it to 165 degrees Fahrenheit or 75 degrees Celsius.

- Label everything with the name of the recipe and the date it was made.

- If the food is frostbitten or has changed color, throw it out.

- Never defrost food and freeze it again. This will trap bacteria in the food and make you very sick.

How to Prep

Now that you have the general guidelines, it's time to go on to more specific meal prepping advice.

Some general principles for meal prep are:

- Choose a specific day each week to do your meal prep. Make sure you do your shopping on the same day so you're working with fresh ingredients. And if you can, get the rest of the family involved too.

- If you've never meal prepped before, start slowly. If you try to prep for every day and every meal on your first try you will probably become overwhelmed. Choose one meal for the first week, like dinner, and start there. You can always expand your prep as you get better at it.

- Buy sturdy containers to store the food in. You may want to freeze the food or heat it up in the microwave, so make sure the containers are safe to use in both appliances.

- Choose recipes you already know. It's very difficult to meal prep a recipe that you aren't familiar with. Try it first, make sure you know what you need and how it should taste. And then you can try preparing it ahead of time.

- Label everything. Write down what's in the containers and the date you made it. If you do this, you won't end up finding mystery containers in your freezer a few months down the track.

- Consider different prep options. There are many different ways to prep. You might want to cook entire meals, separate them into portions, and put them in the freezer. You could just prepare ingredients and box them up ready to eat, or you could just cook a big pot of soup and heat it up as needed. It's all up to you.

- Shop with a list. This might seem pretty basic, but you'd be surprised by how few people actually do it. Before you do your prep, go through your recipes and make a list of everything you need. And don't deviate.

- Remember that it doesn't have to be perfect. It's fine to make mistakes or to throw out a meal because it didn't end up right. You need to find your own way of prepping, and making mistakes is all part of the process.

- And enjoy the time you save!

About the Paleo Diet

Meal prep is particularly good when you're on a specific type of diet. It allows you to eat correctly without having to make complicated meals after a long day at work.

The paleo diet is based on the foods that humans evolved to eat. It's basically a return to the ancient past, and is meant to be a healthier and a more natural way to eat.

Not very long ago in evolutionary terms, humans ate mostly meat, fish, vegetables, fruit and some nuts and seeds. Their digestive systems evolved to eat these foods, and coped well with them.

But then humans started to grow grains and today the modern diet is full of different types of grains. This change has come about quickly, which means that the human body hasn't been able to adjust properly.

Digesting grains effectively and properly is very different to digesting meat, and the human body just isn't equipped to do it.

As a result, a lot of people have developed gluten intolerances or just found themselves gaining more and more weight despite their attempts to diet.

The Paleo diet is an attempt to return to these ancient roots. It's based on the foods that humans evolved to eat.

So processed foods, foods based on grains, and fast foods definitely aren't on the list. And neither are any foods that contain cereals, dairy products, legumes or refined sugar.

Eating like this can be a little hard to do in the modern world. Unfortunately, most pre-prepared foods and even sauces and soups contain ingredients that aren't a part of the Paleo diet.

The Benefits of the Paleo Diet

Once you start eating Paleo, you will enjoy a number of benefits. These include:

- Your diet will be free of additives, preservatives and many chemicals that are part of the modern diet.

- You will probably be eating more vegetables, fruits and nuts, which contain lots of essential nutrients that are often missing from the modern diet.

- If you have food sensitivities, it's likely that your digestion will be smoother and easier on this diet.

- You'll be eating more iron.

- Because the Paleo diet is based on meat, you'll feel fuller between meals and less likely to overeat.

- You may lose some weight because of the food limitations.

Disadvantages of the Paleo Diet

The Paleo diet can be very beneficial for some people. However, there are a number of disadvantages to eating this way including the following:

- It can be expensive because you're eating a lot of meat.

- Most people eat more meat than their body needs these days, and the Paleo diet may exacerbate this problem.

- Products such as grains and dairy products have health benefits that benefit the body, and these foods are banned on the Paleo diet.

- If you're vegetarian, it's very difficult to go Paleo as beans aren't allowed on this diet.

- If you're an athlete or exercise a lot, you need carbohydrates to fuel your muscles and you would need to eat a lot of fruits and vegetables to get the right amount.

- You may experience deficiencies if you take away certain foods and don't replace them properly.

What you can Expect on the Paleo Diet

Changing from the modern diet to a Paleo diet isn't easy, and you should expect some problems when you're just starting out. When people make this change they usually complain about the following side effects:

- Lack of energy: This is probably because you're not eating enough, or because there are less carbohydrates in the Paleo diet. Make some adjustments to the amount you're eating.

- It takes too much time: Eating and cooking Paleo means you have to look for ingredients that match your eating plan and cook from scratch. This can take a lot of time, which is why meal prep can be so helpful.

- Rashes: If you've suddenly added new foods to your diet such as coconut products, this may be the cause of any rashes you notice.

- Digestive symptoms: This is usually because the Paleo diet contains a lot of vegetables. These days, people don't eat nearly enough vegetables, and suddenly changing that can have consequences.

    Try easing up a little on the vegetables and allow your stomach time to adjust. Eventually, you'll be able to eat all the vegetables you want without any problems.

The Paleo diet can easily be adapted into a meal prep routine.

In fact, doing meal prep will help you stick to the diet even on the days when you're tired or just want something fast to eat without stopping at a drive thru.

So with all that in mind, let's learn how to meal prep on the Paleo diet!

Week 1

Breakfast – Banana Granola

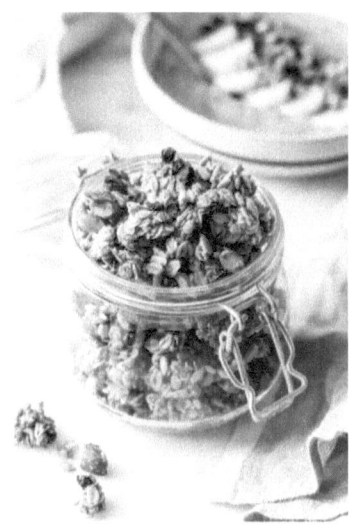

Ingredients

- 1 cup raw walnuts, roughly chopped
- 1 cup of raw cashews, roughly chopped
- 2 medium bananas, ripened and mashed
- 1 cup shredded or desiccated unsweetened coconut
- 1/2 cup sunflower seeds
- 1/2 cup pumpkin seeds
- 2 teaspoons cinnamon
- 1 teaspoon nutmeg
- 2 tablespoons honey
- 1/4 cup melted coconut oil, melted
- 2 teaspoons vanilla extract

Method

1. Heat the oven to 350°F/180°C. Line a baking tray with baking paper. Combine the seeds, coconut, chopped nuts, nutmeg and cinnamon in a mixing bowl.

2. Mash the bananas in a second bowl. Stir in the coconut oil, honey and vanilla extract. Combine the contents of the bowls and mix well.

3. Spread the granola in an even layer on the baking tray and bake for 30-35 minutes. Stir the granola halfway through. When it's golden brown, remove and cool before serving or storing.

This is a great recipe to make and store on your prep day. It will last a long time if kept in an airtight container and you can eat it dry or with a splash of almond milk. This recipe makes 9 servings, so it will easily last you all week.

Lunch – Butternut Squash Soup

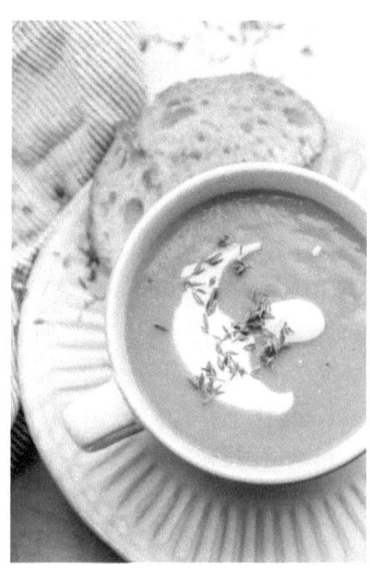

Ingredients

- 4 pears, peeled and diced
- 1 white onion, diced
- 4 cups butternut squash, cubed
- ½ tsp. grated nutmeg
- 1 tsp. dried parsley
- 1 tsp. ginger
- ½ cup coconut cream
- 2 Tbsp. olive oil
- Chives for garnish

Method

1. Add the squash, pears, onions, spices and oil to a pot and bring to a medium heat. Cook for 5 minutes until the onions go clear and add 8 cups of water.

2. Put the lid on and bring to the boil. Reduce and simmer until the squash is soft, around half an hour.

3. Put half the soup in the blender with half of the coconut cream. Blend until smooth. Repeat. Garnish with chives for serving.

This soup will keep well in the fridge and makes 8 large servings. To make it last for the week, set aside 3-4 servings in individual containers and freeze.

Dinner – Paleo Carne Guisada

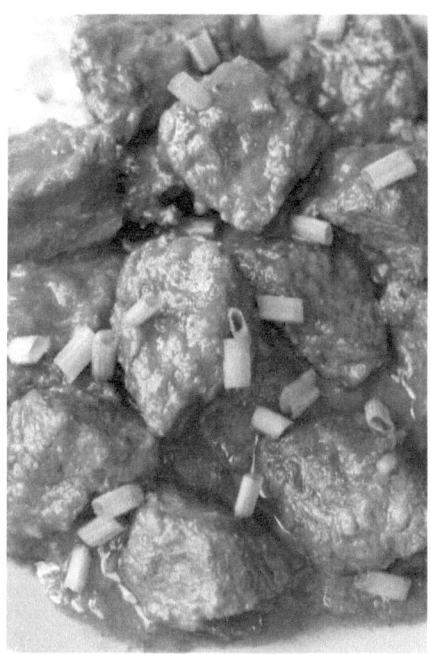

Ingredients

- 4 lbs. beef stew meat, cut into 1" pieces
- 4 cups of beef stock
- 2 medium yellow onions, chopped
- 1 ½ cups of organic tomato paste
- 2 tbsp. cumin
- 4 tbsp. garlic powder
- Ground black pepper
- Pinch of sea salt
- 4 tbsp. Olive oil
- Chopped fresh cilantro, optional for garnish

Method

1. Spread salt and pepper mix over the beef. Heat a heavy pan to medium high heat and brown the beef without completely cooking.

2. Once browned, lower the heat to medium and cook the onion. Add the beef stock, cumin and garlic powder and stir to combine.

3. Add the meat to the slow cooker and pour over the stock. Mix well and cook on low for 6-8 hours or high for 4-5. Serve or freeze and store.

This meal freezes well, so you can easily put 3-4 servings into separate containers and freeze them so you have enough for the entire week. This recipe makes about 8 servings.

Week 2

Breakfast – No Oatsmeal

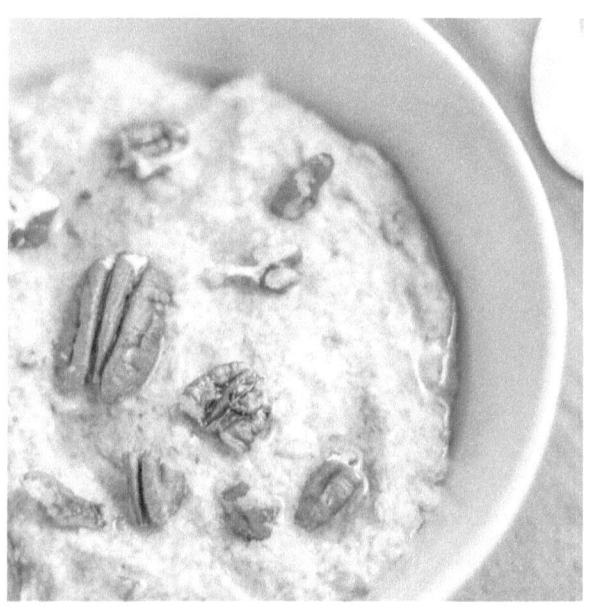

Ingredients

- 1/2 cup sunflower seeds
- 1/2 cup whole flax seeds
- 1/2 cup almonds
- 1/2 cup pecans
- 1/2 cup pumpkin seeds
- 1/2 cup chia seeds
- 1/2 coconut flakes
- 1 cup full fat coconut milk
- 1/2 teaspoon of ginger
- 1/4 teaspoon of nutmeg

- 1 teaspoon of cinnamon
- 1 teaspoon of vanilla
- A pinch of sea salt

Method

1. Pulse all ingredients in the food processor until the pieces are the size of oats. Store and eat.

This will make about 12 servings of oatmeal without using oats, so you can store it in the fridge and eat it for at least a week.

Lunch – Sweet Potato and Bacon Soup

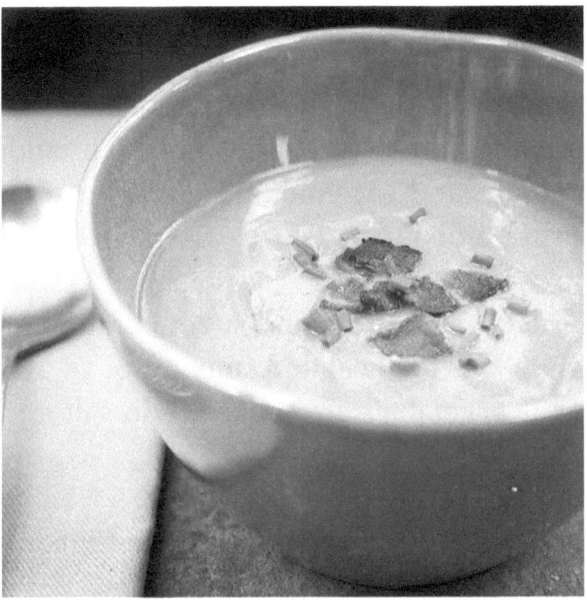

Ingredients

- 8 cups chicken broth
- 6 large sweet potatoes, peeled and roughly chopped
- 2 medium, diced onion
- 8 cloves of minced garlic
- 1 tsp salt
- ½ tsp. pepper
- ½ tsp ground coriander
- Pinch of cayenne
- 1 tsp cumin
- 8 slices bacon

Method

1. Cook the bacon until crisp and set aside on a towel lined plate. When cooler, crumble into pieces. Put 2 tablespoons of the bacon fat into a large saucepan on medium heat. Add the garlic, onion, coriander, pepper, salt, cumin and cayenne and cook for 5-7 minutes or until the onion is soft.

2. Add the chicken broth and sweet potatoes and bring to a boil Reduce the heat and simmer for 15-20 minutes or until the vegetables are cooked. Add salt and pepper to taste.

3. Put the mix into the blender until smooth. Serve garnished with bacon. If you're not eating it immediately, store the bacon separately.

This soup is warm, filling and delicious. You can take it to work in a thermos or other container and heat in the microwave. Add the bacon after reheating.

If you're eating the soup all week at lunch, save half of the bacon to cook later. It will fry up quick and still taste great. This recipe makes about 8 servings.

Dinner – Chicken Curry with Sweet Potatoes

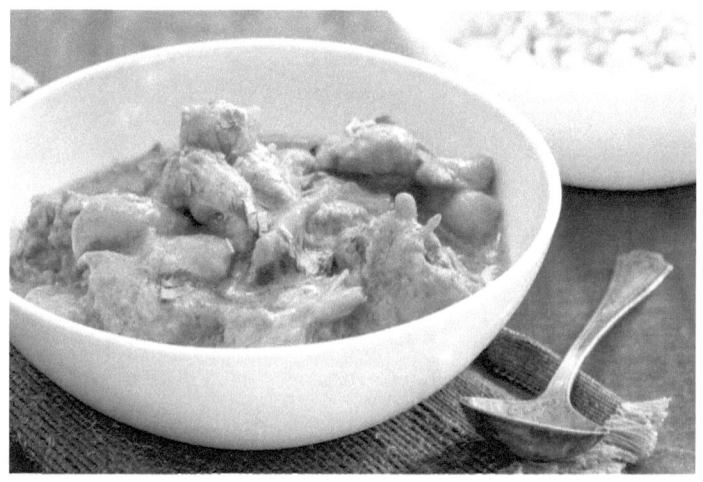

Ingredients

- 16 boneless, skinless chicken thighs
- 2 small onions
- 2 medium cauliflower
- 2 medium sweet potato, peeled and diced into cubes
- 2 head rainbow chard, ribs removed and cut into pieces and leaves sliced.
- ½ tsp cayenne
- 6 tbsp. curry powder
- 6 cloves of minced garlic
- 8 tsp grated ginger
- 2 tbsp. dried coriander
- 2 tbsp. cumin
- 2 bottle 680 mL tomato puree
- ½ tsp sea salt

- 2 400ml cans of lite coconut milk
- 6 tbsp. extra virgin olive oil
- 1 cup frozen shelled edamame (optional)
- sea salt and cayenne pepper to taste
- Pinch each of salt and pepper
- cilantro for garnish
- quinoa (optional)

Method

1. Heat oil in a skillet over medium heat. Season the chicken with salt and pepper and sear on both sides until golden. Set aside.

2. Add another teaspoon of oil to the pan and cook the onion until soft. Add the curry, ginger, cumin, cayenne, garlic, coriander and the salt and pepper and stir until fragrant.

3. Add the tomato puree and the sweet potatoes, cover and simmer until mostly cooked, around 10-15 minutes.

4. Put the chicken thighs in the pan, cauliflower, coconut milk and chard stems. Season with salt and pepper, replace the lid and simmer until the vegetables soften and the chicken is cooked.

5. Remove the lid and stir in the edamame and chard leaves. Cover the pan again until the chard leaves wilt. Serve with quinoa.

This recipe makes at least 8 large servings. Store in the fridge and reheat as needed or freeze part of it for a quick midday meal anytime.

Week 3

Breakfast – Spicy Salmon Frittata

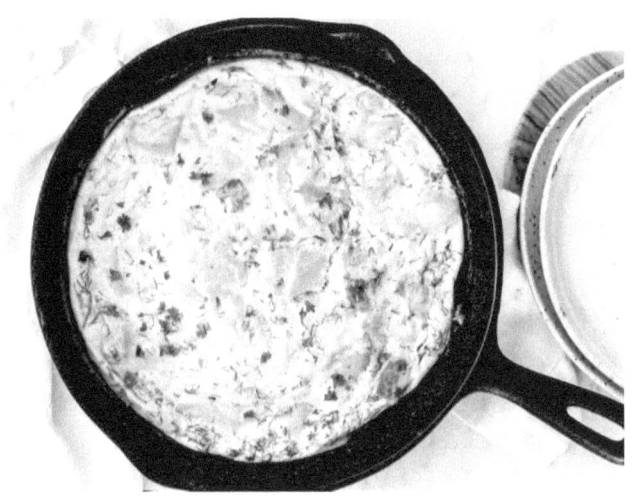

Ingredients

- 1/2 cup wild canned salmon
- 6 soy free eggs, beaten
- 1 Tbsp coconut oil
- 1/2 cup coconut milk
- 1 green pepper, chopped
- 1/2 onion, chopped
- 2 garlic cloves, minced
- 1.5 cups cherry tomatoes
- 2 Tbsp cilantro, chopped
- 1 tsp cumin
- 1/2 tsp paprika
- Sea salt and pepper to taste

Method

1. Preheat the oven to 350 degrees Fahrenheit or 175 degrees Celsius. Melt the coconut oil in a pan then add the onion and the green pepper and cook until soft. Add the garlic. Add the paprika, cumin, salt and pepper.

2. Once the vegetables have cooked down add the tomatoes. Cook the tomatoes for a few minutes and sprinkle in the salmon.

3. Combine the eggs and milk and pour into the pan. Stir well. Cook for a few minutes, adding more salt and pepper to taste. Put the pan in the oven and cook for 15m. Serve with cilantro.

This recipe makes a lovely big pan that's perfect for a week of breakfasts. Just cover and put in the fridge and cut off a nice big slice each morning.

You can also freeze the frittata if you're worried about how well it will keep in the fridge. Eat this meal cold, or warm it in the microwave.

Lunch – Seasoned Turkey Meatballs

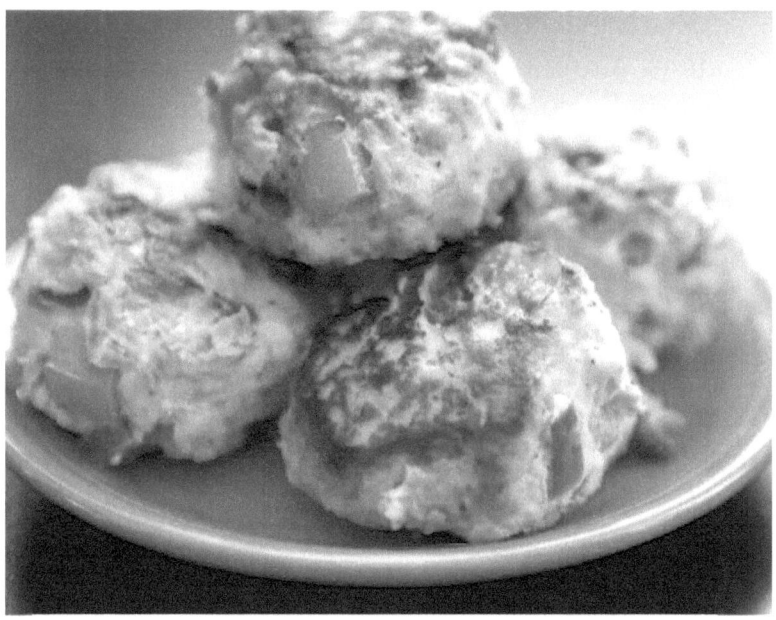

Ingredients

- 2 lbs. ground turkey
- ½ medium, chopped purple onion
- 1 small, chopped red bell pepper
- 2 eggs
- 1 small, chopped green bell pepper
- ¼ cup almond flour
- 1 teaspoon dried parsley
- 3 garlic cloves, finely diced
- 1 teaspoon black pepper
- 1 teaspoon sea salt
- Coconut oil

Method

1. Heat the oil in a pan on medium heat and cook the onions until they're soft. Add the peppers to the skillet and cook for 3 minutes. Add the garlic and cook for a further 3 minutes. Pour the mix into a bowl and set aside.

2. In a second bowl, combine the eggs, turkey, almond flour, sea salt, black pepper and the onion mix.

3. Put some baking paper down on the counter. Take handfuls of the mix and mold them into small meatballs. Line them up on the paper and continue until the mixture is gone.

4. Heat a pan to medium, add the oil and cook 6 meatballs at a time with the lid on. Cook each batch for about 4 minutes on one side.

5. After 4 minutes, turn the meatballs, close the lid and cook for another 4 minutes. Eat hot or seal in the fridge and heat later to eat.

This mixture should make about 20 meatballs. Freeze half of the meatballs so they're safe to eat later in the week and make sure you reheat them properly before eating. You can eat the meatballs alone or with a vegetable mix.

Dinner – Honey Sesame Chicken with Broccolini

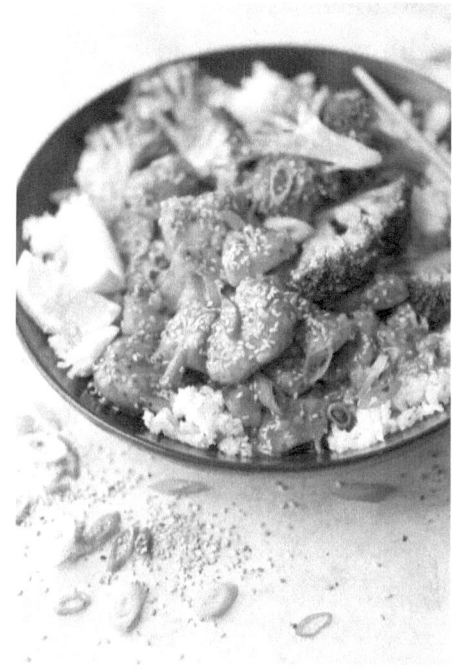

Ingredients

- 1 pound chicken thighs with skin
- ⅓ cup chicken broth
- 2 garlic cloves, minced
- 3 tablespoons soy sauce
- 1 tablespoon sesame oil
- 3 tablespoons honey
- 1 tablespoon fresh ginger, grated
- 1 tablespoon vegetable oil
- Sea salt and freshly ground black pepper

Ingredients for the Sides

- 2 bunches broccolini, ends trimmed
- Cooked Cauliflower Rice
- 1 bunch scallions, thinly sliced
- 1 tablespoon sesame oil
- 2 tablespoons sesame seeds
- Kosher salt and freshly ground black pepper

Method for the chicken

1. Heat the oven to 425 degrees. Season the chicken with salt and pepper. Mix the other chicken ingredients together in a bowl.

2. Heat the oil in an oven-safe skillet over medium heat. Put the chicken in the skillet skin down and sear about 5 minutes until brown.

3. Turn the chicken and add the broth mix. Simmer for 2 minutes on medium high. Take off the heat and put the pan into the oven. Cook about 15-17 minutes or until the chicken is completely cooked.

Method for the sides

1. Combine the broccolini, sesame oil and salt and pepper.

2. Lay the ingredients on a baking sheet and put in the oven once the chicken is done. Roast 8-10 minutes.

3. Split the chicken, broccolini and cooked cauliflower rice between 4 containers and refrigerate.

This recipe makes 4 servings that will keep for four days in the fridge. To make it last throughout the week, double the recipe size. Cook one batch and keep the other until the middle of the week.

Week 4

Breakfast – Vegan Turmeric Protein Donuts

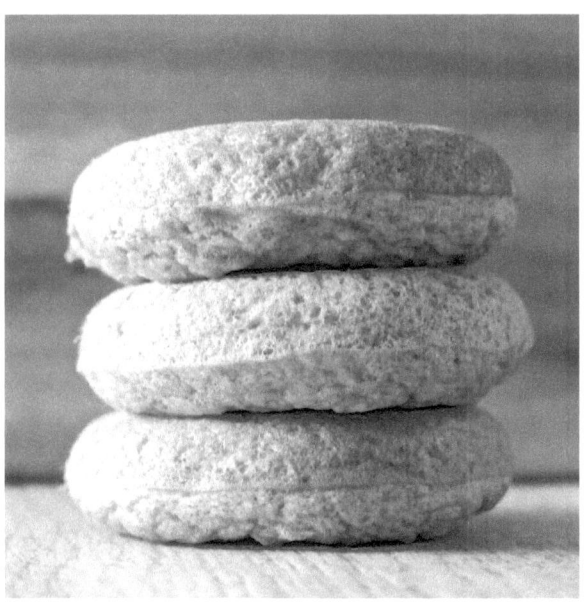

Ingredients

- ½ a cup of pitted Medjool dates
- 1 ½ cups cashews, raw
- 2 tsp. maple syrup
- 1 tsp. turmeric powder
- 1 Tbsp. vanilla protein powder
- ¼ of a cup shredded coconut
- ¼ of a tsp. vanilla essence
- ¼ of a cup dark chocolate

Method

1. Mix all the ingredients except for the chocolate in a food processor and mix on high until the dough is smooth and sticky.

2. Roll the dough into 8 balls and press into a donut mold. Cover the mold with plastic and put in the freezer for 30 minutes.

3. To melt the chocolate, bring a saucepan of water to the boil and place a smaller saucepan on top. Put the chocolate in the pan and stir gently until it's completely melted.

4. Remove the donuts from the freezer and remove from the molds, drizzle the chocolate on top. Store in a container in the fridge.

This recipe will make 8 donuts and will last well in the fridge as long as the container is well sealed.

Lunch – Spinach and Leek Soup

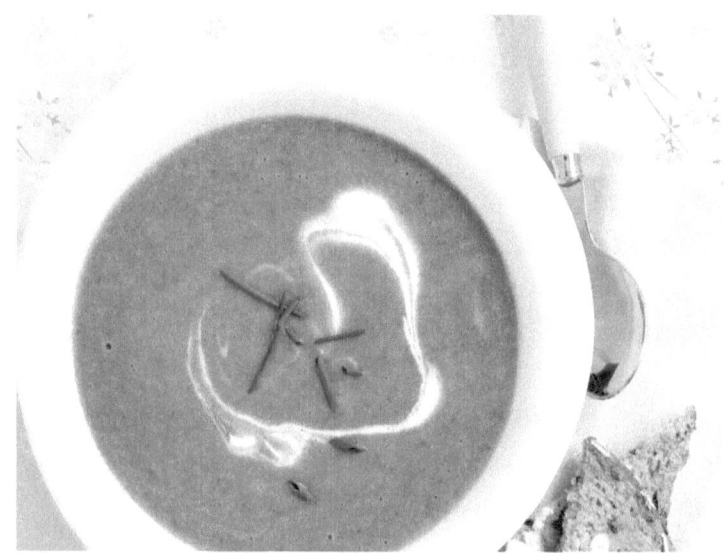

Ingredients

- ½ small head of cauliflower, roughly cut
- 4 sticks celery, roughly chopped
- 2 medium heads of broccoli with stem, roughly cut
- 2 leeks, white parts only, roughly cut
- 2 large handfuls of baby spinach leaves, roughly cut
- 8 cups vegetable stock
- 2 tbsps. ghee
- pinch of ground nutmeg
- 3–4 cloves garlic, roughly cut
- freshly ground black pepper, to taste
- 1 large handful flat-leaf (Italian) parsley, roughly cut
- 1 tablespoon coconut cream (or dairy cream), to garnish
- drizzle of truffle oil, to garnish (optional)

Method

1. Heat the ghee over medium in a pot, add the garlic and leeks until the leeks are soft. Add the broccolini, cauliflower and celery and cook for 5 minutes.

2. Add the vegetable stock, bring to the boil and then lower the heat and simmer for 10-15 minutes until the vegetables are cooked. Take off the heat and add the spinach and parsley.

3. Blend the soup until smooth, add the pepper and nutmeg to taste. Serve hot with nutmeg cream and optional truffle oil.

This recipe makes at least 7 servings of soup, so you can keep a few servings in the fridge for lunch and freeze the rest for later.

To make the meal even heartier, add some shredded cooked chicken while heating.

Dinner – Turkey Chili

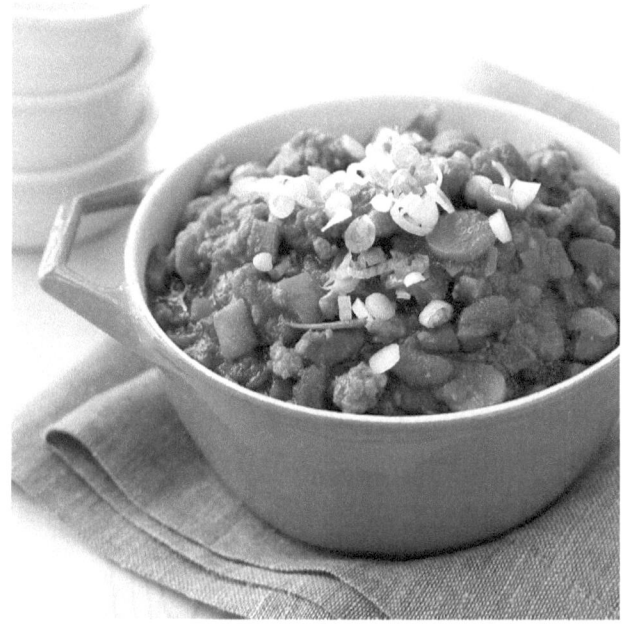

Ingredients

- 2 lbs ground turkey
- 1 cup chopped carrots
- 1 cup chopped peppers
- 40 oz can of crushed tomatoes
- 1 cup onion, minced
- 1 tbsp garlic, minced
- 1 ½ paprika
- ½ tsp. cinnamon
- ½ tsp. turmeric
- 1 tsp. cumin
- ½ tsp. salt
- 2 tsp. chili powder

- 1 tsp. pepper
- 1/2 tsp. red pepper flakes
- 2 tbsp olive oil

Method

1. Heat the oil and cook the turkey until it's browned.

2. Add all the ingredients and the turkey to the slow cooker and stir well. Cook on low for 6 hours.

This recipe makes about 8 servings, so it will last you an entire week in the fridge or you can freeze it to enjoy later.

Conclusion

Eating a good diet, one that's healthy and full of the foods that nourish and support your body, is absolutely vital if you want to be healthy and happy.

Unfortunately, this isn't as easy as it sounds these days. If you have a busy life, the lure of ready-made meals can be too much for you on the days when you're tired and just need something fast.

This is when you might end up eating foods that are highly processed, full of fats and salt, and sadly lacking in nutrients.

But now there's another option. No matter what type of diet you're on, learning how to do meal prep can greatly reduce the amount of time you spend cooking food on a day to day basis.

With your pre-prepared meals in the fridge, you will be able to cook food that suits your Paleo diet in just a fraction of the time it would normally take you.

This can be an absolute lifesaver on busy days and nights, and you'll be able to enjoy all the great health benefits that come with sticking to your eating plan without sacrificing other activities.

So give meal prep a try, and watch your busy nights become more organized, happier, and healthier.

Final Words

I would like to thank you for purchasing my book and I hope I have been able to help you and educate you on something new.

If you have enjoyed this book and would like to share your positive thoughts, could you please take 30 seconds of your time to go back and give me a review on my Amazon book page.

I greatly appreciate seeing these reviews because it helps me share my hard work.

You can leave me a review on Amazon.com.

Again, thank you and I wish you all the best!

www.ingramcontent.com/pod-product-compliance
Lightning Source LLC
Chambersburg PA
CBHW021134080526
44587CB00012B/1277